Table of Contents

Introduction

Collagen, the essential skin protein. The invisible support structure keeping skin firm, plump and young from the inside-out and the outside-in.The protein whose decline is regulated like a timer. Every year, from our late twenties, skin will lose it at a rate of 1%* (1) since its production slows down. But this happens even faster if we over-eat foods that accelerate this natural 1% decline.

To find out how much the foods that pass our lips impact the collagen in our skin, read on.

Collagen is protein molecules made up of amino acids. It provides structural support to the extracellular space of connective tissues. Due to its rigidity and resistance to stretching, it is the perfect matrix for skin, tendons, bones, and ligaments.

Collagen can be further divided into several groups depending on the type of structures they form. There are 28 various types of collagen that have been discovered, but by far, the most common are types I through IV, with type I comprising over 90% of the collagen in the human body.

Collagen type I is the most abundant protein in mammals. It confers mechanical stability, strength and toughness to a range of tissues from tendons and ligaments, to skin, cornea, bone and dentin. These tissues have quite different mechanical requirements, some need to be elastic or to store mechanical energy and others need to be stiff and tough. This shows the versatility of collagen as a building material. While in some cases (bone and dentin) the stiffness is increased by the inclusion of mineral, the mechanical properties are, in general, adapted by a modification of the hierarchical structure rather than by a different chemical composition. The basic building block of collagen-rich tissues is the collagen fibril, a fiber with 50 to a few hundred nanometer thickness. These fibrils are then assembled to a variety of more complex structures with very different mechanical properties. As a general introduction to the book, the hierarchical structure and the mechanical properties of some collagen-rich tissues are briefly discussed. In addition, this chapter gives elementary definitions of some basic mechanical quantities needed throughout the book, such as stress, strain, stiffness, strength and toughness.

When collagen levels drop

Collagen is a protein — the most plentiful protein in your body. It's in your muscles, bones, tendons, ligaments, organs, blood vessels, skin, intestinal lining and other connective tissues.

While you can't measure your collagen level, you can tell when it's falling. Collagen decreases as you get older, contributing to:

- Wrinkles and crepey skin
- Stiffer, less flexible tendons and ligaments
- Shrinking, weakening muscles
- Joint pain or osteoarthritis due to worn cartilage
- Gastrointestinal problems due to thinning of the lining in your digestive tract

Aside from aging, the top reason people don't have enough collagen is poor diet. "Your body can't make collagen if it doesn't have the necessary elements.

Making collagen naturally

When your body makes collagen, it combines amino acids — nutrients you get from eating protein-rich foods, like beef, chicken, fish, beans, eggs and dairy products.

The process also requires vitamin C, zinc and copper. You can get vitamin C by eating citrus fruits, red and green peppers, tomatoes, broccoli and greens. You can get the minerals by eating meats, shellfish, nuts, whole grains and beans.

As you age, however, your body may no longer absorb nutrients as well or synthesize them as efficientlys. To make sure your body has enough ingredients to make collagen, you may need to change what you eat or take dietary supplements.

The best collagen-boosting food

In addition to healthy servings of foods packed with protein, vitamins and minerals.You can buy it in grocery stores or make it yourself.

Bone broth draws collagen out of beef, chicken or fish bones, leaving a flavorful liquid that you can drink straight up or use in other dishes. Most bone broth recipes require slowly simmering bones in water — on the stove or in a crockpot for one or two days.

I recommend buying only organic bone broth, or cooking broth from the bones of only organically raised animals. You don't want the residue of pesticides, antibiotics and other contaminants in your broth.

Second best: collagen supplements

If you're eating a healthy diet and feeding your body all the nutrients it needs to make collagen, you probably don't need a supplement, Dr. Bradley says. But there's nothing wrong with taking one.

Hydrolyzed collagen (or "collagen peptide") powder usually has no flavor and dissolves easily in beverages, smoothies, soups and sauces.

As for skin cream with synthetic collagen, it may work. It will add a film-like layer to your skin to reduce water loss and act as a barrier from environmental elements. But using skin cream is probably not as effective as healthy eating and protecting your skin from excessive sun exposure and sunburns, especially early in life.

Your skin is your body's largest organ. The same way you nourish collagen stores throughout your body will nourish your skin too.

Collagen

You probably think about collagen in your skin because the word comes up whenever anyone is talking about skin aging. It's true that this protein plays a role in the perceived youthfulness of your skin, but there's more to it. Collagen is a protein and is one of the main building blocks of our skin. It's also found in our bones, tendons, and ligaments.

Time for a fun fact: Collagen makes up 75 percent of skin's support structure. Think of collagen as the frame of your mattress; it gives [your skin] structure and support. To continue with the mattress analogy, the springs are elastic fibers and the stuffing is hyaluronic acid.

Which Factors Contribute to the Loss of Collagen in the Skin?

Unfortunately, collagen starts to degrade with age, and your genetics can affect how fast that degradation happens. We lose collagen year after year, and make lower quality collagen. Free radicals damage collagen they are our skin's enemy. Environmental factors (like UV rays or pollution), bad lifestyle habits (smoking), and a poor diet (for example one high in sugar) all create free radical formation, which speeds collagen breakdown.

Let's hit on smoking for a moment. One of the best things you can do for your skin is never smoke or quit smoking if you do.

Research suggests that smoking allows free radicals to attack collagen fibrils, rendering them weak and of poor quality. It's not surprising, therefore, that the skin of a smoker tends to look damaged and wrinkled, particularly around the mouth.

Foods That Help Your Body Produce Collagen

- Bone broth
- Chicken
- Seafood
- Egg whites
- Citrus
- Berries
- Tropical fruits
- Garlic
- Leafy greens
- Beans
- Cashews
- Tomatoes
- Bell peppers
- Keep an eye on sugar

Can supplements replace foods?

To supplement or to eat?

Diet plays a surprisingly large role in the appearance and youthfulness of your skin. And that all comes down to collagen.

Collagen is the protein that gives skin its structure, suppleness, and stretch. There are many types of collagen, but our body mainly consists of type 1, 2, and 3. As we age, we produce less collagen in our skin every year — hence the tendency toward wrinkles and thinning skin we see the older we get.

This explains the boom of collagen supplements touted in our social feeds and store shelves these days. But are collagen pills and powders the best route? The key difference between the two may be down to the bioavailability the body's ability to use a nutrient.

Why you should consider food first

Foods like bone broth contain a bioavailable form of collagen your body can use right away, making it arguably superior to supplements.

Eating collagen-rich foods or foods that boost collagen production may also help create the building blocks (amino acids) you need for your skin goals. There are three amino acids important for collagen synthesis: proline, lysine, and glycine.

1. Bone broth

While recent research finds bone broth may not be a reliable source of collagen, this option is by far the most popular by word of mouth. Made by simmering animal bones in water, this process is believed to extract collagen. When making this at home, season the broth with spices for flavor.

Since bone broth is made of bones and connective tissue, it contains calcium, magnesium, phosphorous, collagen, glucosamine, chondroitin, amino acids, and many other nutrients.

However, each bone broth is different because of the quality of the bones used along with other ingredients.

To guarantee the quality of your broth, try making your own with bones obtained from a reputable local butcher.

2. Chicken

There's a reason why many collagen supplements are derived from chicken. Everyone's favorite white meat contains ample amounts of the stuff. (If you've ever cut up a whole chicken, you've probably noticed how much connective tissue poultry contains.) These tissues make chicken a rich source of dietary collagen.

Several studies have used chicken neck and cartilage as a source of collagen for arthritis treatment.

3. Fish and shellfish

Like other animals, fish and shellfish have bones and ligaments made of collagen. Some people have claimed marine collagen is one of the most easily absorbed.

But while your lunchtime tuna sandwich or dinnertime salmon can certainly add to your collagen intake, be aware that the "meat" of fish contains less collagen than other, less desirable parts.

We don't tend to consume the parts of fish that are highest in collagen, like the head, scales, or eyeballs. In fact, researchers have used fish skin as a source for collagen peptides.

4. Egg whites

Although eggs don't contain connective tissues like many other animal products, egg whites do have large amounts of proline, one of the amino acids necessary for collagen production.

5. Citrus fruits

Vitamin C plays a major role in the production of pro-collagen, the body's precursor to collagen. Therefore, getting enough vitamin C is critical.

As you probably know, citrus fruits like oranges, grapefruit, lemons, and limes are full of this nutrient. Try a broiled grapefruit for breakfast, or add orange segments to a salad.

6. Berries

Though citrus tends to get all the glory for its vitamin C content, berries are another excellent source. Ounce for ounce, strawberries actually provide more vitamin C than oranges. Raspberries, blueberries, and blackberries offer a hefty dose, too.

Furthermore,berries are high in antioxidants, which protect the skin from damage.

7. Tropical fruits

Rounding out the list of fruits rich in vitamin C are tropical fruits like mango, kiwi, pineapple, and guava. Guava also boasts a small amount of zinc, another co-factor for collagen production.

8. Garlic

Garlic may add more than just flavor to your stir-fries and pasta dishes. It could boost your collagen production, too. According to Gabriel, Garlic is high in sulfur, which is a trace mineral that helps synthesize and prevent the breakdown of collagen.

It's important to note, however, that how much you consume matters. "You probably need a lot of it to reap the collagen benefits.

But with its many benefits, it's worth considering garlic part of your regular diet. If you love garlic, take the measurement in a recipe and double it.

Is there such a thing as too much garlic?

Garlic is safe in regular amounts, but too much garlic (especially raw) may cause heartburn, an upset stomach, or increase your risk for bleeding if you use blood thinners. Avoid eating more garlic just for collagen purposes.

9. Leafy greens

We all know leafy greens are a key player in a healthy diet. As it turns out, they may offer aesthetic benefits, too.

Spinach, kale, Swiss chard, and other salad greens get their color from chlorophyll, known for its antioxidant properties.

Some studies have shown that consuming chlorophyll increases the precursor to collagen in the skin.

10. Beans

Beans are a high-protein food that often contain the amino acids necessary for collagen synthesis. Plus, many of them are rich in copper, another nutrient necessary for collagen production.

11. Cashews

Next time you reach for a handful of nuts to snack on, make it cashews. These filling nuts contain zinc and copper, both of which boost the body's ability to create collagen.

12. Tomatoes

Another hidden source of vitamin C, one medium tomato can provide up to almost 30 percent of this important nutrient for collagen. Tomatoes also boast large amounts of lycopene, a powerful antioxidant for skin support.

13. Bell peppers

While you're adding tomatoes to a salad or sandwich, toss in some red bell peppers, too. These high-vitamin C veggies contain capsaicin, an anti-inflammatory compound that may combat signs of aging.

Sugar and refined carbs can damage collagen

To help your body do its best production of collagen, you can't go wrong with high-collagen animal or plant foods or vitamin and mineral-rich fruits and vegetables.

And if you don't like the foods listed, remember there's no one source. A diet full of protein-rich foods, whether from plant or animal sources, can help supply these critical amino acids.

Other nutrients that aid the process of collagen production include zinc, vitamin C, and copper. So, fruits and vegetables high in vitamins and minerals are also a friend to supple skin.

And, for even more dramatic results, be sure to stay away from too much sugar and refined carbohydrates, which can cause inflammation and damage collagen.

Some critical questions about collagen and diet

Sometimes a variety of foods is hard to consistently get in your diet. And some have questioned whether consuming collagen-rich foods actually translates to firmer skin. It's possible that stomach acid may break down collagen proteins, preventing them from reaching the skin.

And since dietary collagen for anti-aging is still a relatively new area of research, many experts hesitate to draw definite conclusions.

Still, some research does look promising. A 2014 double-blind study published in the journal Skin Pharmacology and Physiology found that women who consumed extra collagen had higher levels of skin elasticity after four weeks than those who took a placebo.

Another study observed a 13 percent reduction in the appearance of lines and wrinkles in healthy females after 12 weeks on a collagen supplement.

That said, collagen isn't only for smooth, elastic skin. Collagen may also help with joint pain, muscles, or digestion. So, if collagen supplements sound more accessible to your routine and wallet, we say it's worth a try.

Can eating collagen stop skin ageing?

Collagen was once best known as an injection to plump lips and soften lines. But the beauty industry has found a tastier, less painful way for you to get your fill. Collagen powders, bars, chocolates, chews and liquid and capsule supplements are some of the products claiming to support your body's collagen levels and keep signs of skin ageing at bay.

If you're tempted by this seemingly tasty fountain of youth, let's ask the question… what on earth is collagen and does eating or drinking it really keep your skin looking younger for longer?

Why are people eating and drinking collagen?

Collagen is the glue that holds your body together. We have lots of types of collagen, but most is Type-I, which is the main structural protein in skin.

Type-I collagen gives skin shape and strength, but starts to break down faster than your body can replace it in your mid-20s. At this age, skin begins to lose thickness and strength at a rate of around 1.5 percent a year.

Collagen has long been a popular ingredient in skin creams, but there is a question over whether it can penetrate the epidermis (outer layer of skin). Injecting collagen has fallen out of favour, as it doesn't last as long as some alternative fillers and has been associated with complications such as allergic reactions.

An increasing number edible collagen-containing products are appearing in the shops. Flavourings and sweeteners are often added to make them more appealing. You can also buy unflavoured collagen powder to stir into juices, smoothies, soups and even coffee.

What types of collagen are we eating?

There are two kinds of collagen used in edible products: whole and hydrolysed.

Whole collagen is broken down into peptides (amino acids, the building blocks of protein) during digestion in the gut, "just like any other protein", says dietitian Sophie Medlin. It's claimed these peptides make their way to your skin dermis (an inner layer of skin, containing blood vessels, nerves and hair follicles), replacing or topping up your collagen levels.

Hydrolysed collagen is already broken down into peptides before it is consumed. One theory is this fools your brain into thinking that damage has been done to your collagen, spurring your body to produce more.

Collagen is found in and therefore often derived from animals such as cows, pigs and fish or other seafood. Products containing collagen are not vegetarian and may be unsuitable for people with other dietary requirements.

Does eating or drinking collagen work?

Some studies support the effectiveness of eating hydrolysed collagen on improving hallmarks of skin ageing by inducing collagen production, improving skin elasticity and increasing hydration and collagen density in the skin.

Recipes

Paleo "Candy" Sour Gummies

Yields: approx 30 gummies

6 blood oranges + 3 meyer lemons (or approximately 3 cups liquid)

2 limes, juiced

pinch of salt

6 tbsp. Vital Proteins Collagen Protein Gelatin

(2 tbsp. gelatin is needed for every 1 c. of liquid used)

Directions:

Peel the oranges and lemons, discard the peels, and place the entire fruit into a blender. Add the lime juice and a pinch of salt. Blend on high speed for 1-2 minutes or until the mixture is very smooth. (Optional: juice the fruit instead to have a sweeter, less sour gummy. Be sure to check the total amount of liquid used to keep your liquid to gelatin ratio consistent).

Pour half the mixture into a small saucepan, add the gelatin, and stir very well with a whisk. Heat over low heat until the mixture is warmed (not hot) and the gelatin has mostly melted, about 3-5 minutes max. CAUTION: leaving the mixture over too hot of heat will quickly activate the gelatin and cause your mixture to turn into a thick sludge.

Pour the warm mixture back into the blender and blend again until smooth, about 30 seconds. Then portion the liquid into silicone ice cube molds (like these shown above) or any baking dish (you can cut them yourself). Refrigerate for 2+ hours before removing and consuming, this will give enough time for the gelatin to solidify the gummies. Keep refrigerated up to 2 weeks.

Homemade Orange Jello

Ingredients:

2 cups orange juice

2 T. great lakes gelatin (where to buy gelatin)

Directions:

Pour 1/2 cup of orange juice into saucepan on low heat.

Pour in your gelatin and mix well until disolved.

Pour in the remaining juice and turn off heat.

Pour into gelatin into a glass bowl.

Let cool and place in the fridge for at least 3 hours.

Enjoy!

HOMEMADE LEMON GUMMY BEARS

What you will need to make your own healthy gummy bears:

1/3 cup fresh squeezed lemon juice

3 Tbsp grass fed gelatin (where to get quality gelatin)

2 Tbsp raw honey (where to get quality honey)*

Directions:

Pour lemon juice and honey into a skillet on low heat- not hot since it will kill the probiotic awesomeness of the raw honey!

Once warm mix in the gelatin.

Mix thoroughly until the gelatin has dissolved.

Pour into a measuring cup, and then into molds (we used these super cute bear ones and heart ones)

Put in freezer for 15 minutes.

Take out and enjoy!

Strawberry Lemon Kombucha Gummies

Lemon Panna Cotta

INGREDIENTS

1 can full fat coconut milk (like this), divided

1 and 1/2 tsp grass fed gelatin (like this)

3 TBS raw honey (like this) OR real maple syrup (like this)

zest from 2 lemons

1 tsp vanilla extract

OPTIONAL: lemon zest for garnish

INSTRUCTIONS

Whisk together one cup of the canned coconut milk and lemon zest in a medium pan. Bring to just below a boil, turn off heat, cover, and allow to infuse.

Pour the rest of the coconut milk into a shallow bowl and sprinkle the gelatin evenly over the surface and allow to BLOOM for 10 minutes.

Once gelatin has bloomed, gently reheat the coconut milk/lemon mixture to just below a boil and whisk in the coconut milk/gelatin until completely dissolved. Turn off heat.

Whisk in the sweetener of choice and vanilla.

Strain with a sieve and pour into 3 small dishes and allow to chill until set (at least 4 hours.)

Run a sharp knife around the edge of each cup and unmold onto a serving plate, and garnish as desired OR you can place the chilled cups into a hot water bath for a minute or two to make removal a titch easier.

NOTES

I usually use a canned coconut milk without any additives. However, I have found that this panna cotta tends to separate a bit if there are no emulsifiers in it. It still tastes AMAZING. It just isn't as pretty.

Salted Caramel Fudge

Ingredients

1/4 cup Tinstar Food's brown butter ghee (or) non-hydrogenated palm shortening for AIP

1/4 cup coconut oil

1/4 cup Vital Protein's collagen powder

2 tbsp maple sugar (or) stevia for Keto

1 1/2 tsp maca powder (omit for AIP)

1 1/2 tsp vanilla powder

1 tbsp coconut flour

1/2 cup shredded unsweetened coconut

1/2 tsp sea salt

Process

In a food processor, puree the first six ingredients together until smooth.

Next, either pulse in the shredded coconut until broken down (or) mix it in by hand to keep it in shredded form.

Scoop the mixture into desired candy molds or a standard loaf pan lined with parchment paper, then stick whichever container you use into the freezer to allow the fudge to set.

Maple Pumpkin Collagen Shake

I always have frozen bananas to hand, they're perfect for whipping up an impromptu ice cream or shake. Whenever I notice the ones on the counter top are turning a little on the over ripe side, into the freezer they go!

(makes 2 large or 4 small)

1/2 cup pumpkin puree (I use this one)

juice 1 large navel orange

1 cup (250ml) coconut milk (I use this one)

2 frozen bananas, peeled and roughly chopped

1 tbsp maple syrup (I use this one) *

1/2 tsp cinnamon (I use this one)

2 tbsp collagen hydrolysate (I use this one)

pinch sea salt (I use this one)

Put all ingredients into a blender and whizz until completely smooth and well blended, adding a dribble or two of filtered water if you find it too thick. Serve immediately.

Sunbutter Chocolate Collagen Protein Bars

instructions

In a food processor, combine the sunflower seeds, coconut flakes, and coconut oil. Process until a smooth butter forms. This will take 5-10 minutes.

Scrape the coconut sunbutter into a bowl and add the collagen peptides, maple syrup, salt, and vanilla. Mix well.

Form the mixture into a 1/3 inch thick rectangle on a parchment-lined baking sheet. Freeze for a few minutes.

Meanwhile, make the coating: to a small microwave-safe bowl, add all the coating ingredients. Microwave a few seconds, just until melted, and stir.

Use a knife to cut the the sunbutter and coconut rectangle into bars. Then coat them in chocolate. I did this by spreading a thin layer of coating on a plate, then placing the bar on top and spooning the coating over the top of the bar to cover. Then transfer the bars back to the baking sheet and pour the rest of coating over them.

Freeze just until set, then store in an airtight container in the fridge.

Orange Cranberry Collagen Gummies

Ingredients

2 Scoops NeoCell Beauty Infusion - Tangerine

1 C. Cold Water

1 C. Cranberry Juice

6 Tbsp. Unflavored Gelatin Powder

Instructions

Mix your scoops of your beauty infusion into the cold water until it is dissolved.

Sprinkle your gelatin over the beauty infusion mixture slowly one TBSP at a time. Stirring inbetween. It will be very thick and somewhat gritty.

Heat your cranberry juice until it barely begins to boil.

Mix your orange gelatin mixture into the hot cranberry juice stirring until all lumps are dissolved.

Remove from heat and pour into molds.

Place in fridge until they set then remove from molds. Keep them covered.

If you would still like making them but you don't have any Beauty Infusion, you can just use orange juice. You may need to add some Stevia or something of the like for added sweetness as well.

Bone Broth Latte

Ingredients

1 mug bone broth (beef or chicken) heated to a boil

1+ tablespoons Organic Coconut Oil (unrefined)

1+ tablespoons Organic Grass-Fed Butter or Ghee

2 scoops collagen for an additional 18 grams of protein

Optional Ingredients:

1+ tablespoons mct oil use in place of coconut oil

Instructions

Combine hot broth, coconut oil and butter in your blender and (carefully) blend on high for 20 seconds.

Paleo Protein Cookie Dough

INGREDIENTS

2 medium Japanese sweet potatoes, peeled and chopped into ½ inch pieces (about very 2 heaping cups)

¾ cups canned coconut milk, recommended brand available here

1 Tbs. coconut butter, recommended brand available here

1 Tbs. coconut flour

1 Tbs. coconut sugar, maple syrup or raw honey (optional)

1 tsp. vanilla extract

3 scoops Vital Proteins Collagen, available here

Pinch of salt

¼ cup chocolate chips (dairy/soy free option available here)

INSTRUCTIONS

Steam the peeled/chopped sweet potatoes until tender, about 15-20 minutes. Let cool.

In a food processor, blend the sweet potatoes with the remaining ingredients (except the chocolate chips) until creamy.

You are welcome to make the happy mistake I made when I first made the recipe. I added the chocolate chips while the dough was slightly warm, and they got all melty and soft and yummy. But the result wasn't as pretty with bleeding chocolate chips. So if you don't want the chocolate to melt, make sure the mixture is cool before stirring in the chocolate chips.

Enjoy or store in the fridge for a few days.

Paleo Strawberries & Cream Collagen Bar

INGREDIENTS

2 cups large flaked unsweetened dried coconut

1 cup raw cashews

¾ cup dried strawberries

2-3 tablespoons coconut cream

3-5 tablespoons coconut oil, melted

⅓ cup collagen peptides

1 teaspoon pure vanilla extract

2 tablespoons coconut flour

¼ teaspoon sea salt

INSTRUCTIONS

In a food processor, combine the coconut and cashews. Process until a smooth butter forms, scraping down the sides as needed.

Add the strawberries and process until combined.

Transfer to a large mixing bowl and stir in remaining ingredients (will be thick).

Press into a glass 8"x8" baking dish. Freeze until set but not frozen.

Cut into bars. Store in an airtight container in the refrigerator.

Raw Cacao Mint Shake

Ingredients

8 ounces full fat coconut milk or any other raw or non-dairy milk

1/4 cup avocado

1 to 2 tablespoons cacao powder

1 to 2 tablespoons raw honey to taste

1 tablespoon sustainably sourced collagen (certified glyphosate free)

6 to 8 dried peppermint fresh

1 to 2 tablespoons allergy-friendly chocolate chips optional, but yummy!

1/2 cup ice cubes made from pure water

Instructions

Combine ingredients in the order listed in a blender.

Blend until smooth and enjoy!

Recipe Notes

*Don't have fresh mint? Use 1 to 2 drops peppermint essential oil instead.

Whipped Coconut Pudding

Ingredients

1 cup additive-free coconut milk

4 tsp gelatin

1 Tbsp honey (see notes above for alternatives)

1/4 tsp ground ginger (for spiced version only)

1/8 tsp ground cardamom (use cinnamon for AIP--optional; for spiced version only)

1/8 tsp ground nutmeg (omit for AIP--optional; for spiced version only)

Instructions

In a small bowl, stir together ¼ cup coconut milk and the gelatin. This ensures the gelatin dissolves without clumps.

Heat the remaining coconut milk in a small saucepan. When simmering, whisk in the softened gelatin mixture. Whisk until dissolved.

Place in the fridge until set, at least 4 hours.

When gelatin is set, scoop it out into a food processor or blender.

Add the sweetener of your choice and the spices. Pureé until creamy, about 2-3 minutes.

Taste and adjust sweetener/spices, if needed.

No-Bake Cookie Dough Bites

Ingredients

1/2 cup Organic Gemini Tigernut flour

1/2 cup Vital Protein Collagen Peptides

2/3 cup shredded coconut

1/4 cup coconut oil

1/4 cup maple syrup

1/4 tsp sea salt

2-4 tbsp chocolate (or) carob chips

1 tsp vanilla extract

Process

In a medium sized mixing bowl, sift together tigernut flour, collagen powder, shredded coconut, and sea salt.

In a separate bowl, whisk together vanilla, maple syrup, and coconut oil, then pour it over the dry ingredients, mixing with a spatula until just combined, then fold in the chocolate chips.

Use your hands (or) a cookie scoop to form 12 like-size cookie dough bites, placing each one on a parchment lined plate.

Once through with making all 12 bites, place the plate in the freezer and allow to chill for atleast 30-40 minutes until the coconut oil has solidified.

Store the treats in the freezer or fridge and remove when ready to eat.

Paleo Chocolate Coconut Smoothie

Ingredients

1 cup coconut milk

1 frozen banana sliced

1 cup ice

1/4 cup raw cacao powder

1 scoop collagen protein powder

Instructions

Add all ingredients to Vitamix or high power blender and blend until smooth.

Nutrition

Calories: 160kcal | Carbohydrates: 23g | Protein: 2g | Fat: 8g | Saturated Fat: 7g | Cholesterol: 0mg | Sodium: 86mg | Potassium: 375mg | Fiber: 5g | Sugar: 7g | Vitamin A: 40IU | Vitamin C: 5.1mg | Calcium: 14mg | Iron: 1.6mg

Melon Gummies

Ingredients

3 cups ripe melon, cubed

1/4 cup water

3-4 TB raw honey

1/4 cup grass-fed gelatin

Instructions

Put the cantaloupe and water in a small sauce pan and bring to a simmer. Stir for a few minutes while everything warms.

Turn off the heat and add the raw honey. Stir to combine/melt.

Put the warmed melon mixture in a food processor or blender, add the gelatin, and blend completely.

Pour into your silicone molds (this amount fills about 48 slots in my molds) and refrigerate. I like to stick them in the freezer to make this part go faster – only takes about 15 minutes or so! The firmer, almost frozen gummies pop out of the molds nicer/easier too!

After the mixture gels up, you can pop out the gummies – I just push the silicone mold "inside-out" – works great!

Store your gummies in the fridge. They keep fine in the lunchbox without an ice pack though!

Bulletproof Coffee Gummies

1 cup hot fresh brewed organic coffee

1 TBSP grass fed butter

1TBSP Organic coconut oil

1TBSP organic vanilla extract

5 TBSP grass fed gelatin

Sweeten to taste with stevia, honey or maple syrup

Blend all in your blender until mixed well and frothy. Pour into candy molds and put in the fridge until set (time varies from 20 minutes to 2 hours). Pop out of the molds and store in a baggy or jar until you are ready to eat them. These travel very well and provide a quick energy boost along with healthy fats and protein!

Pumpkin Pudding with Gelatin

Ingredients:

15 oz (1 can) full-fat coconut milk

1/3 cup pureed canned pumpkin (or make your own!)

1 Tbsp honey (preferably raw)

1 Tbsp gelatin

1 tsp vanilla extract

½ tsp cinnamon

Directions:

Add all ingredients (excluding the gelatin) to a small pot and warm on low/med heat

Use an immersion blender to blend ingredients

Add gelatin and mix again with the immersion blender

Turn off heat and pour into container to cool

Put in fridge for 1 hour

Enjoy!

Coconut Flour Pancakes with Gelatin

INGREDIENTS

¼ cup coconut flour, a free bag from Thrive is available here

1 Tbs. grassfed gelatin, available here

4 pastured eggs, at room temperature

1 heaping Tbs. softened butter or coconut oil

½ cup canned coconut milk

Coconut oil or ghee, for the pan

INSTRUCTIONS

Start heating a seasoned cast iron skillet or enamel skillet over medium heat. Whisk together the coconut flour and gelatin. Stir in the eggs, beating until a smooth paste forms.

Stir in the butter/coconut oil until combined, then add the coconut milk.

Cook the pancakes in the hot skillet with coconut oil/ghee. Cook until the edges and center starts to look opaque, then flip. Smaller pancakes will be easier to flip.

Cherry Ginger Gummies

INGREDIENTS

3 tablespoon lemon juice

¾ cup water

1 cup fresh or frozen cherries

¼ cup maple syrup

1 teaspoon powdered ginger

¼ cup gelatin

INSTRUCTIONS

Pour lemon juice, water, and cherries into blender and blend on high until smooth.

Pour mixture into saucepan. Turn heat to medium-low and whisk in maple syrup, ginger, and gelatin. Continue to whisk for 5 minutes, until the mixture is thin and there are no clumps.

If using a mold, place mold on baking sheet for ease of transfer to refrigerator. Carefully pour mixture into mold or baking dish. Set in refrigerator to firm for 1 hour.

If using a mold, transfer to freezer for 5 minutes (set a timer!) in order to easily pop gummies from the mold. If using a baking dish, cut into squares.

Cake Batter Collagen Protein Bars

INGREDIENTS

½ cup coconut butter, available here or here

¼ cup + 1 Tbs. grassfed collagen, also known as collagen hydrolysate (not gelatin), available here

1 Tbs. honey or maple syrup

1 Tbs. coconut oil

½ tsp. vanilla extract or ⅛ tsp. pure vanilla bean powder, available here

Pinch of salt

INSTRUCTIONS

The coconut butter should be soft enough to stir. Like coconut oil, the consistency of coconut butter varies with the room temperature. If it is solid, I recommend placing the jar in a pan of hot water, allowing the water to come halfway up the sides of the jar. Sit for 5 minutes to soften, then stir until creamy.

Line a baking sheet with unbleached parchment paper or have ready a silicon mold such as this one.

Note on the sweetener: depending on what sweetener you use, the consistency of the bars will vary slightly. If you use stevia, for example, the batter may be too liquid to create a free-form square on the parchment paper. You may need to divide the mixture into the wells of a silicone mold, then chill.

In a bowl, combine the coconut butter and collagen. Add the honey. When the honey is added, the mixture will become slightly crumbly.

Add the coconut oil, which will help "pull together" the mixture. If necessary, add another teaspoon or two of coconut oil.

Add the vanilla and a pinch of salt.

Transfer the mixture to the baking sheet and form into a square with your hands. Score the square with a knife to create small bars. Chill in the fridge until firm, about 30 minutes. Then cut into bars along the scored marks.

Store in an airtight container in the fridge. If desired, let soften slightly at room temperature before eating.

Healing Hot Chocolate

Ingredients:

1 can full fat coconut milk

14 ounces water (I refill the coconut milk can)

3 tablespoons maple syrup

1/4 teaspoon Vitamin C crystals (333mg per serving)

3 heaping tablespoons Gelatin (1 tablespoon per serving)(omit for Vegan option)

3 drops of 1000 iu Vitamin D drops (1000iu per serving) or THIS ONE for Vegan option

heaping tablespoon organic cocoa powder

Optional: 1 teaspoon Unflavored Magnesium Powder (can be a little tart for some so omit if concerned)

Optional: 10 drops Chocolate Stevia Drops

Combine all ingredients in a pot over high heat and whisk until well combined – the cocoa powder should be completely dissolved

Split into 3 mugs and serve right away

Chocolate Sweet Potato Pie

Ingredients

½ cup dates

2 cups walnuts preferably soaked and dehydrated

4 sweet potatoes baked and peeled

½ cup cocoa powder

⅛ teaspoon unrefined salt

¼ cup ghee could sub coconut oil or butter

7 tablespoons honey just short of ½ cup

¼ cup cold water or cold coffee, for extra intensity

2 tablespoons gelatin powder

250 g strawberries approximately 14 medium, or 9 oz.

sweetener of choice to taste

2 tablespoons water

1 tablespoon gelatin powder

Instructions

Crust:

Blend dates in food processor until the dates are in small pieces.

Add nuts and process until mixed.

Distribute clumps of dough around a pie plate, then use your hands to flatten and spread evenly on the bottom and up the sides.

Chill.

Chocolate Filling:

Sprinkle gelatin over water and let sit.

Blend sweet potatoes, cocoa powder, and salt in a food processor or blender.

Melt ghee and honey in a small pot (double boiler is ideal).

Add the water/gelatin mix and stir until dissolved and immediately take it off heat. Don't let it boil or the gelatin won't set.

Pour the warm liquid into the cocoa mixture as the machine is running.

Process until well mixed, pour into crust.

Chill.

Strawberry Gelee:

Sprinkle gelatin in water.

Puree strawberries in a food processor or blender until smooth.

Add sweetener until desired sweetness is achieved (this will depend on the sweetness of your strawberries. I used about 1 Tbsp of honey)

Warm water/gelatin in double boiler until dissolved, immediately add to strawberry puree while machine is running.

Pour gelee mixture on top of semi-set chocolate filling.

Chill the pie until set, about 5 hrs in the fridge.

Cut and to serve to enjoy a slice of silky smooth goodness!

Notes

This recipe requires chilling between steps.

Green Tea, Lemon & Ginger Gummies

Ingredients

3/4 cup / 180 ml cold water

5 tablespoons grass fed gelatin powder

1/2 cup strongly brewed green tea (I used 4 of these bags)

6 tablespoons ginger juice

1/4 cup lemon juice

Optional, to taste: raw honey

Instructions

BLOOM: Pour the water into a saucepan. Sprinkle the gelatin powder over the surface of the water and allow to dissolve. Set aside.

BREW: Make the tea in accordance with instructions for steeping time. Remove tea bags and make sure you have 1/2 cup brewed tea.

DISSOLVE: Add the brewed tea, ginger juice and lemon juice to the saucepan with the bloomed gelatin. Gently warm the saucepan and stir until all the gelatin has dissolved and there are no lumps. Do not overheat. If you're adding honey, do that now.

CHILL: You can pour the gelatin mixture into molds (like the one I used) or into a baking dish. Refrigerate for at least 2 hours to set before trying to remove them from a mold or cut them into pieces.

Notes

These gummies are Autoimmune Paleo compliant.

Using this adorable gingerbread man silicone mold, I got about 20 large ginger gummies. You can make them in whatever molds you like, or simply pour the mixture into a baking dish and then cut into pieces once it has set.